Reproduction or translation of any part of this work beyond what's permitted by Section 107 or 108 of the 1976 United States Copyright Act without permission of the copyright owner is unlawful. Requests for permission or further information should be addressed to the author.

This publication is designed to provide accurate and authoritative information in regard to the subject matter covered. It is sold with the understanding that the publisher or author does not render legal advice. If legal advice or another expert assistance is required, the services of a competent professional should be sought.

The Truth About ICD-10
Printed in the United States of America

ISBN-13: 978-1503201262
ISBN-10: 1503201260

© 2015. All rights reserved.

No part of this book or accompanying materials may be reproduced by any mechanical, photographic, or electronic process, or in the form of a photographic or audio recording. No part of this book may be stored in any retrieval system, transmitted, or otherwise copied or circulated for public or private use without prior written permission of Nitin Chhoda.

The author and publisher make no representations or warranties with respect to any information offered or provided in this book regarding effectiveness, action, or application of the protocols contained herein. The author and publisher are not liable for any direct or indirect claim; loss or damage resulting from the use of the information contained herein.

We are at the cusp of the biggest challenge and the biggest opportunity in healthcare.

TABLE OF CONTENTS

CHAPTER 1

What Everyone is Afraid Of 1

Transition Codes in October 2015 - New Coding Options 2

Greater Latitude 2

Major Changes 3

CHAPTER 2

Why ICD-10 Will Benefit Everyone 5

Codes for the New Era 5

Identifying Fraud, Trends and Abuse 6

Grading Performance 6

Improved Analytics for Practitioners 7

CHAPTER 3

Breaking the Code 9

CHAPTER 4

The Power of Ten 11

Ten Things to Know to Prepare for ICD-10 11

1 – ICD-10 Scheduled to Replace ICD-9 in October 2015 11

2 – The Change Is Mandatory and Inevitable 12

3 – ICD-10 Codes will Impact Everyone 12

4 – Your EMR Should be Able to Map ICD9 > ICD10 > SNOMED Codes 13

Crosswalk Determination 13

SNOMED Concept ID(s) 14

5 – Early Preparation Is Critical 15

6 – CPT Codes Will Stay the Same 16

7 – Identify Any Needed Documentation Changes 16

8 – Make the Conversion a Top Priority 16

9 – Be Prepared for an Emergency 17

10 – Invest in Education for your Staff 17

CHAPTER 5

Three Biggest Mistakes to Avoid With the ICD-10 Transition 19

Substantial Decline in Productivity 19

Billing Staff Considerations 20

Complacency (The Notion that 'It Will Get Delayed') 20

CHAPTER 6

Implementing Your Preparation 23

Where to Get Assistance 23

Creating a Strategic Planning Team 24

Budgeting and Planning 24

Communication between Staff and with Vendors is Critical . 24

Testing Your Level of Preparation for ICD-10 25

Documentation and Coding Principles May Need Modification 25

CHAPTER 7

The Countdown Begins..................27
Conduct an Impact Analysis 27
Finding a Vendor 27
Communication is Key..................28
Custom Templates and Modifications 28
Training for Success 28

CHAPTER 8

Reverse Engineering ICD-10 Preparation 31
Create a Contingency Plan 31
Budgets and Deadlines..................32
Communicate With Others..................32
New Rules and Compatibility 32
Education, Skills, and Resources 33
Fix Existing Problems..................33
Acceptance is Key..................33

CHAPTER 9

Are You Ready? 35

CHAPTER 10

The Transition 37
More Codes for All 37
Easing the Transition 38
Training Opportunities..................39
Plan for Contingencies..................39

CHAPTER 11

Minimizing Financial Havoc 41

Maintain Cash Reserves – Plan Ahead 41

Training and Education Essentials – Invest in Resources 42

In-House or Outsourced Billing – Examine Pros and Cons ... 42

The Impact of Security Vulnerabilities – Protect Data 43

Prepare for the Threat of RAC Audits – Maintain Compliant Documentation 43

CHAPTER 12

Implementing EMR for ICD-10 45

Get your team used to using hardware 46

Analyze your workflow 46

Input all data 46

Upgrade to the necessary hardware 47

Assign a Project Manager or Team Leader 47

Include Everyone 48

Invest in Training Programs 48

Be Flexible 49

CHAPTER 13

EMR Implementation to Improve Workflow and Cash flow 51

Some of the benefits include: 51

Easy Access to Records 52

Compliant, Comprehensive Documentation 53

Rapid Transmission of (and Access to) Medical Records 53

Streamlined, Efficient Billing 54

Legibility of Information 54

How to Choose... 55

Focus on Design.. 55

Analytics is Important.. 55

Avoid Gimmicks and Sales Pitches 56

An EMR Can Lead to Personal Freedom 58

Verifying Insurance Coverage 58

Fewer Hours and More Money 58

24/7 Access 59

Space and Time.. 59

Errors and Reimbursements.. 59

Resources

Programs For Healthcare Professionals 63

Software For Healthcare Professionals 67

Schedule A Call 72

About The Author 75

Index 79

THE TRUTH ABOUT ICD-10

CHAPTER 1

What Everyone is Afraid Of

On October 1, 2015, ICD-10 will officially be implemented. Adjusting from the old system of coding to the new system can be stressful and frustrating without the right preparation and appropriate software to rely on.

A lot has changed since the implementation of ICD-9.

ICD-10, which is scheduled to replace ICD-9 in October 2015 will impact healthcare professionals throughout the country.

New diseases have emerged, a better understanding of old ailments is available, and advances in treatment have made the old codes obsolete.

Healthcare professionals have been struggling for years trying to code for treatments and services that didn't quite fit the range of possibilities available through the new techniques and technology. That's all going to change when the switch to ICD-10 happens.

Transition Codes in October 2015 - New Coding Options

The good news is that several thousand new coding options will be introduced into the current system of 13,600, making it easier for practice owners to bill for new treatments and procedures.

While it opens up multiple opportunities for clinics, the number of new codes for ICD-10 will wreak havoc with practices without the right electronic medical record (EMR) software. ICD-10 is going to be the first major coding update since 1977, and it's going to take the medical field by storm.

The ICD-10 codes represent the 10th update of the International Statistical Classification of Diseases and Related Health Problems (ICD).

Greater Latitude

The upcoming changes in coding offer healthcare providers greater latitude when submitting reimbursement claims and providing treatments. The deadline for implementation has been pushed back many times.

The most recent delay, from October 1, 2014 to October 1, 2015, was partly instituted to allow those in the healthcare field to establish an EMR in their practice to facilitate the use of the new codes.

ICD-10 CODES are significantly different from the old codes. They range from 3-7 digits in length and are used for documenting a diagnosis. An EMR will make the transition considerably smoother but will still require extensive planning and staff training.

To add another level of difficulty to the transition, before healthcare providers can use the new coding, they need to implement HIPAA's 5010 transaction standards. Claims for reimbursement that don't use the ICD-10 codes after the deadline will face rejection.

Major Changes

The changes in coding affect healthcare providers and impact insurance companies and how practice owners get reimbursed. The ICD-10 codes reflect changes in all facets of healthcare, from new diseases and vaccines to medications and treatments.

The changes allow healthcare professionals to code in greater detail and offer more specific details about each diagnosis. The coding allows clinicians to provide new services and offers more opportunities to be paid, but clinic owners should expect the changes to be disruptive at first.

In a world of international travel, where pandemics are a real concern, the new ICD-10 codes will be an essential tracking tool. They will assist authorities to track contagious and potentially devastating diseases. These include various types of flu, HIV and AIDS, along with different forms of cancer. In particular, this will help the World Health Organization and the Center for Disease Control.

ICD-10 codes represent an update that's long overdue.

The new coding allows for a greater range of diagnosis and is required if therapists are to be reimbursed for their treatments and services.

The first ICD codes were developed by Jacques Bertillon in 1893 in France and adopted by the U.S. in 1898.

Technology and healthcare knowledge have improved steadily throughout subsequent decades, and the latest incarnation of the ICD codes provides healthcare professionals with the tools to manage patient care and the profitability of their practices more efficiently.

CHAPTER 2

Why ICD-10 Will Benefit Everyone

ICD-9 codes were originally designed as a classification system to compile statistics, but as a code set, ICD-9 does not provide the information that payers desire for reimbursements or the type of data needed to monitor situations like disease outbreaks. This is important for entities like the Centers for Disease Control (CDC) and the World Health Organization (WHO).

In other words, it is now an outdated code set.

Implementation of the new code set is mandatory, and there are a number of compelling reasons for the transition, from patient management to identifying and addressing potential pandemics.

The codes were developed by the health division of the United Nations, and the U.S. is one of the last countries to implement the codes -- a move that has been questioned by other nations.

Codes for the New Era

The ICD-9 system is running out of number combinations adequately to describe new diseases and illnesses, terminology and technological advances since its implementation in 1979.

The ICD-10 codes employ an alphanumeric diagnosis and procedural system that is more precise.

ICD-10 is designed to provide significantly more specificity and accuracy. It can (and most likely will) increase the amount of documentation required for reimbursements.

The new system offers the ability to code for new diseases, techniques and procedures as they emerge in the coming years.

Identifying Fraud, Trends and Abuse

The new codes provide additional oversight for payers, allowing them to identify instances of fraud, trends among practitioners, and individuals who are abusing the system. It's a tool that the insurance companies will use to reduce the cost of healthcare.

Grading Performance

The utilization of ICD-10 codes allows payers and professional organizations to monitor how clinicians are utilizing available resources, in an effort to provide better patient care and effective management to reduce overall costs.

The new codes provide payers and government officials with a means to grade the individual performance of healthcare providers and facilities, establish reimbursement rates and set public health policies.

Improved Analytics for Practitioners

The new codes offer analytic tools for clinicians, allowing them to track patient illness, injury and disease trends. Clinicians will have enhanced tools to monitor instances of everything from cancer and domestic abuse to diabetes and obesity rates.

Practitioners have no choice but to transition to ICD-10.

Modifying patient records to reflect the new codes will require a significant investment of time and effort, but many healthcare professionals are looking forward to a change that has the potential to improve patient care.

CHAPTER 3

Breaking the Code

The first image below shows the breakdown of ICD-9 coding to ICD-10 Coding.

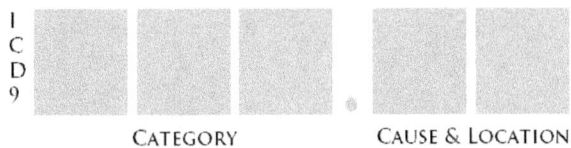

The image below shows two examples of ICD-9 to ICD-10 conversion. The first example shows a one-to-one match for the code. The second shows the additional options for further specificity.

719.7
(Unspecific Joint Disorders: Difficulty Walking)

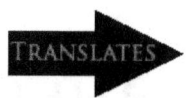

R26.2
(Difficulty Walking, Not Classified Elsewhere)

781.2
(Abnormality of Gait)

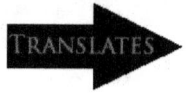

Potential Codes
(R26.0, R26.1, R26.89, R26.9)

CHAPTER 4

The Power of Ten

Ten Things to Know to Prepare for ICD-10

It's essential that practitioners begin preparing now to reduce potential payment problems and delays when the new codes go into effect.

So who does this impact? Does it impact the front desk, the clinician or the biller?

The answer is it impacts every single person in your practice. Those who won't prepare will learn the hard way, and the lessons will reverberate through the staff for a long time.

Here are ten things to know to prepare your practice for the upcoming ICD-10 code switchover on October 1, 2015.

1 – ICD-10 Scheduled to Replace ICD-9 in October 2015

After October 2015, only ICD-10 codes will be accepted for billing and diagnostic purposes. Remember, this applies to the date of service, not to the date of submission of the claim.

So if the date of service is before October 1, 2015 and submitted after October 1, 2015 (and there will be several cases like this in your practice), you'll still use ICD-9 to code those visits.

Any claim with a date of service after October 1, 2015 that doesn't use an ICD-10 code can be automatically rejected, but practitioners can't use the new codes before the official launch date. This is subject to change and it is best to check individual payer guidelines.

The new alphanumeric codes represent the International Classification of Diseases for expanded accuracy.

2 – The Change Is Mandatory and Inevitable

It's a mandatory transition that all clinicians must make if they want to be paid. The codes reflect new diseases, conditions, treatments and technological advances. It's the first update in 30 years, providing clinicians with additional coding tools to diagnose and treat patients.

3 – ICD-10 Codes will Impact Everyone

The new codes affect all healthcare providers, from clinicians to hospitals. Being prepared will minimize delays and denials in payments and ensure that everyone in the office is familiar with the technology being used to implement the change.

4 – Your EMR Should be Able to Map ICD9 > ICD10 > SNOMED Codes

An Electronic Medical Record Software, such as In Touch EMR, will help your practice adapt to this monumental coding change. Sophisticated systems, like In Touch EMR, will seamlessly manage all the new codes, allowing your practice to bill efficiently.

The system you choose must have a crosswalk between ICD-9, ICD-10 and SNOMED codes built in. A system like this will allow you to generate compliant documentation and clean claims, allowing you to maintain or increase cash flow in your practice.

Here's an example of a crosswalk, which should automatically exist in your EMR system. This crosswalk will train and alert your clinicians about ICD-10 and make the transition seamless.

We are going to use the sample ICD-9 code of lumbago, which most rehabilitation professionals are familiar with.

7242 LUMBAGO

Crosswalk Determination

ICD-10 CODE

M545 Low back pain

SNOMED Concept ID(s)

279040009 Mechanical low back pain (finding)

402245001 Angry back syndrome (disorder)

298236009 Lumbar spine stiff (finding)

279039007 Low back pain (finding)

247368002 Posterior compartment low back pain (finding)

301407002 Tenderness of right lumbar (finding)

279041008 Lumbar trigger point syndrome (finding)

278860009 Chronic low back pain (finding)

301408007 Tenderness of left lumbar (finding)

278862001 Acute low back pain (finding)

300957005 Postural low back pain (finding)

279042001 Lumbar segmental dysfunction (finding)

161894002 Complaining of low back pain (finding)

267982002 Pain in lumbar spine (finding)

202794004 Lumbago with sciatica (finding)

As a clinician, you need access to this crosswalk at your fingertips as the countdown towards October 1, 2015.

In fact, your EMR should show you which ICD-9 code corresponds to which ICD-10 and which SNOMED code. This will train your clinicians to understand which ICD-9 codes correspond to which ICD-10 codes right away.

When the big day comes in October 2015, this 'crosswalk capability' in your technology will make your transition seamless. Without this capability, practitioners and billers across the country will be scrambling to adjust to the new changes.

If you don't have a crosswalk like this built into your EMR system, you need to plan ahead. You will need to purchase or identify crosswalk data for the most common ICD-9 codes in your practice. It is good practice for clinicians and office staff to start studying this data right away.

5 – Early Preparation Is Critical

The change over takes place promptly on October 1, 2015 and reflects a one-year delay issued by the Department of Health and Human Services. While that may sound like plenty of time, early training is essential to the process.

Clinicians will need time to install any needed software, train employees, conduct tests and work out any bugs in their system.

An implementation strategy must be developed, along with a timeline and impact assessment evaluation. Practitioners will need to communicate with vendors, clearinghouses and insurance agencies to ensure security and compliance.

6 – CPT Codes Will Stay the Same

ICD codes are for making a diagnosis and current procedural terminology (CPT) codes are for healthcare and rehabilitation billing. The next generation of ICD-10 codes won't affect the use of CPT codes for healthcare services.

7 – Identify Any Needed Documentation Changes

The change to ICD-10 will require clinicians to modify or change their documentation processes. A significant increase in documentation time is expected according to several industry sources. Practitioners using an EMR must have the ability to create custom templates for documentation. Having the flexibility to document in a personalied manner will make it easier to implement any changes required.

8 – Make the Conversion a Top Priority

The change to ICD-10 codes should be a top priority for clinicians across the nation, even though it will require a significant amount of time and effort to ensure the transition goes smoothly.

The change represents a complete overhaul of the coding system, and clinicians that don't invest the time to prepare could run into significant delays in reimbursements or claim denials.

9 – Be Prepared for an Emergency

Part of the conversion process includes a contingency plan in the event that a major problem manifests.

Employees should be cognizant of whom to contact and be able to do so 24/7 to have their office systems up and running again quickly. It is best for practices to have a financial contingency in place in case payments are delayed or paused for a period. A line of credit or access to emergency funds is critical to meet expenses like rent, payroll, and supplies.

10 – Invest in Education for your Staff

The best thing practitioners can do for their practice is to educate themselves and their staff to be informed of any changes relating to the coding change.

Identify and schedule training for anyone within the office that will be directly involved with the billing and coding process. The clinicians and the billers need to identify courses on ICD-10 preparation and study crosswalks by working closely with their EMR vendor. The change to ICD-10 codes is mandatory, affecting everyone in the healthcare industry and the time to prepare for implementation is counting down with each day.

Clinicians have a variety of resources to call upon and should make a concerted effort to ready themselves and their staff for the October 1, 2015 deadline.

Practitioners shouldn't count on another implementation delay because this deadline is not going to be delayed. It's going to happen and all healthcare professionals need to be prepared for it.

CHAPTER 5

Three Biggest Mistakes to Avoid With the ICD-10 Transition

Substantial Decline in Productivity

When Canada implemented ICD-10 codes, it was only a fraction of what the U.S. plans to add on October 1, 2015.

Unfortunately, the outcome in Canada was less than desirable. The problem was that the productivity among physicians and billers/coders was impacted and several clinicians struggled to return to pre-implementation levels.

With ICD-10 implementation, some unpredictable things are likely to occur. The sheer number of codes, combined with the new and unfamiliar alphanumeric code combinations, could dramatically reduce productivity.

That translates into reduced reimbursements and greater turnaround times on claims.

The first few months of implementation will be a critical time for practices financially as they deal with inevitable errors that mistakenly deny claims and require multiple resubmissions, further slowing down the system and cash flow.

Billing Staff Considerations

Experienced billers and coders are in short supply, and those with in-depth knowledge of ICD-10 codes are harder to find.

The problem associated with a lack of awareness of ICD-10 codes will diminish as more people are trained, but the shortage doesn't bode well for practice owners trying to maintain their cash flow.

Complacency (The Notion that 'It Will Get Delayed')

Many practice owners aren't moving as quickly as they should and are preparing sufficiently for the coding transition out of a sense of complacency.

Some are hoping another delay in implementation will buy them more time, while others either aren't sure where to begin or view it as a simple software upgrade.

Some see the coding changes as an inconvenience and not one that's a high priority.

The Centers for Medicare and Medicaid Services has indicated there will be no more delays and the implementation will occur on October 1, 2015 as planned. The organization has an extensive array of data, resources, and timelines to assist practices prepare.

Clinicians that aren't ready on the implementation day will face severe consequences. Any claims with a date of service after October 1, 2015 without ICD-10 codes will automatically be denied. The ICD-10 transition will affect every practice.

Extensive training for staff, electronic medical record software upgrades and hardware systems will be required. The procedure will place added stress on staff, disrupt routine office procedures and affect the financial health of clinics.

Procrastination won't make the ICD-10 transition go away, and it's far better for practices that prepare for the deadline over time instead of waiting until the last minute and hoping for the best.

Clinicians that don't adjust their practices will suffer from reduced productivity and the inability to collect reimbursement claims.

CHAPTER 6

Implementing Your Preparation

There's much to do before the mandatory transition to ICD-10 codes and little time to accomplish a mountain of tasks. Much of the ICD-10 code training plan, enacted by clinicians, will depend upon the size of their practice.

The deadline for the exclusive use of the new codes is on October 1, 2015. It's very unlikely that clinicians will receive another reprieve in the form of yet another nationwide delay.

Where to Get Assistance

Before an implementation strategy can be created, it's essential to know what resources are available that can provide assistance.

The Centers for Medicare and Medicaid Services is a primary resource and has a multitude of data for different sized practices and facilities.

EMR vendors, coding/billing software vendors, and the American Health Information Management Association can also prove helpful.

Creating a Strategic Planning Team

Few practitioners have enough time in the day to treat patients and become ICD-10 experts. Creating a project team will free clinicians to conduct the daily business of the practice and allow them to obtain essential facts upon which to make informed decisions.

Budgeting and Planning

Implementation will affect practices in a variety of ways that include software upgrades, purchasing hardware and manuals and obtaining staff training.

Based upon a comprehensive audit of the clinic's current systems, the project team should create an action plan. This plan should take no more than two months to provide clinicians with the needed data to develop a realistic budget and secure appropriate funding for needed changes.

Communication between Staff and with Vendors is Critical

Communication is an essential ingredient in ICD-10 preparation and it will be an ongoing process. Practitioners will need to inform staff about the changes, how it will affect them, and establish a training schedule that doesn't interfere with the operation of the practice.

Communication extends to all the vendors, payers and clearinghouses with which the practice interacts. Find out when their systems will be in place and when testing can begin.

Glitches in the system can't be avoided, making it imperative for clinicians to monitor other entities to determine their readiness, ensure software systems are compatible and passed performance testing.

Testing Your Level of Preparation for ICD-10

Multiple tests should take place prior to the 2015 deadline. Systems will need to be tested to determine if claims can be submitted, and if documentation can be completed accurately and efficiently. Staff will need to be proficient in their understanding of the new codes and the ways it will affect them.

Documentation and Coding Principles May Need Modification

The forms and documents a practice currently uses may require significant changes or modification, or new templates may need to be created to facilitate the documentation and coding process.

Billers and coders will need in-depth training and extensive practice in the practical application of the codes to avoid claim rejections. They will also need sufficient time to work with any changes in the forms they use to gain proficiency.

Practitioners should be prepared for glitches, errors, and last minute changes among the entities with which they regularly communicate with.

The change to ICD-10 codes represents significant changes in the way clinicians document their patients' complaints, along with the software and systems they use to do so. Being prepared for potential problems demonstrates a realistic and responsible attitude that will help practices survive the ICD-10 storm.

CHAPTER 7

The Countdown Begins

The transition to ICD-10 codes requires preperation.

Practitioners need to prepare now and establish a timeline to give themselves adequate time for staff training, to update/upgrade systems and conduct testing.

Conduct an Impact Analysis

The code transition will affect systems and people in multiple ways. Clinicians will need to conduct an impact analysis to determine how extensively implementation will affect both manual and electronic systems.

The American Medical Association has indicated that the process of updating clinician and vendor systems will take up to six months.

Finding a Vendor

Practitioners will need to contact vendors to ascertain costs and how quickly implementation of new software and hardware can be completed.

It's essential to find a vendor that supports staff training and maintains responsibility for updates/upgrades while minimizing costs. Clinicians may find that they need to locate a new supplier to meet their needs.

Communication is Key

No practice stands alone, and clinicians will need to communicate with one another, their biller or billing service, vendor, clearinghouses and insurance companies, to ensure systems are compatible. Extensive system testing will be required between all the entities involved and will take two to three months to complete.

Custom Templates and Modifications

Clinicians should begin now to familiarize themselves and staff with the new codes. Documentation may need modification to reflect coding changes, create claims and accommodate data collection methods.

Don't use cookie cutter templates – create customized templates that are relevant to the practice.

An EMR and billing software that provide crosswalks between ICD-9 and ICD-10 codes are critical.

Training for Success

Staff training will take two to three months. An efficient training schedule is needed to provide every staff member with a working knowledge of the codes and how it will affect their duties but one that minimizes the effects on daily operations. Providing training exercises using the new codes is a good practice for the implementation deadline.

The transition to ICD-10 codes will not happen overnight. It takes extensive planning and communication between the parties involved.

ICD-10 isn't a catastrophe, but getting caught unprepared will be catastrophic for the survival of practices. A single disruption in the chain could result in lost revenue and practices going out of business.

CHAPTER 8

Reverse Engineering ICD-10 Preparation

The change to ICD-10 codes will impact a host of office systems and software, along with the human element of practices. Glitches and errors with implementation are inevitable, and the objective for the practice should be to minimize issues with the transition.

Claims will be affected by a project of this scope. Clinicians will have to do well in their preparations beginning with the anticipated outcome and do so as if they were facing a natural disaster.

Create a Contingency Plan

To overcome the upcoming storm of the ICD-10 transition, practitioners should create a comprehensive list of monthly expenses that includes their bills and payroll. Plan on putting aside at least three months worth of cash to cover expenses in the event that the reimbursement flow decreases.

Budgets and Deadlines

Practitioners will face a multitude of expenses in the form of staff training, software and office system upgrades. Practices must establish a timeline to accomplish their goals, from where and how staff will receive training to when software and hardware will be installed. If problems occur, clinicians will know where the delays are, allowing them to adjust their plans accordingly.

Communicate With Others

Everyone, from payers, vendors, and clearinghouses, must comply with the implementation of the new codes. To assist clinicians with their project deadlines, it's a good idea to talk with others in the practice's network to discover when each entity plans to have their systems in place so testing can begin.

New Rules and Compatibility

It's critical for clinicians to identify the top 10 ways the transition will affect their practice. Some payers, such as those for Workers' Compensation, may be exempt from the change and this varies from one state to another. It's best to speak direcly with your payors for more information.

Practitioners will have to conduct due research to ensure they have a system that's compliant and compatible with clearinghouses and payers.

Education, Skills, and Resources

Staff will need sufficient time to be trained on the new alphanumeric codes, their usage and how they will affect their daily duties. Compile a list of resources the office and staff can utilize. It's never too early to begin the familiarization process.

Coding is a specialized field, and some clinicians may find that hiring a biller/coder who already has expertise with the new codes is more cost-effective for the practice.

Fix Existing Problems

Before attempting software installations and upgrades, identify and fix any problems with existing systems, software, and processes. Problems anywhere within current systems and practices will create even more difficulties later on.

Acceptance is Key

ICD-10 implementation is mandatory, and the U.S. is one of the last countries in the world to adopt the system. Each practice should have a designated person to become an expert on all the nuances, rules and regulations of ICD-10.

That individual will be a key element in the creation and development of an implementation program that's compliant, compatible and helps guard reimbursement reflections.

Sufficient preparation for implementation will reduce stress throughout the practice and ensure that claims are reimbursed promptly. It's understandable that clinicians are anxious about the change to ICD-10 codes, but with only a little while to go before the codes are in common use, practitioners have no time to waste.

CHAPTER 9

Are You Ready?

Use the following checklist to review if you have secured your practice and staff as "ICD-10 Ready".

Who do I contact for software issues?

_____

Who is the point-person or Team Leader in my practice?

_____

When was my last test of my clinic to see if all forms and workflow were ICD-10 ready?

_____

CHAPTER 10

The Transition

While ICD-10 is not a phased change in the industry, your practice's transition should be.

Many clinicians describe the change to ICD-10 codes as exciting, but others use words that include scary and expensive. Training in the use of the new codes will be required for many employees, especially for coders/billers, which has many in the profession viewing the change with trepidation.

The American Health Information Management System (AHIMA) has determined that it will require about 16 hours and $500 to train coders working in a small practice. This assumes that these individuals have prior experience with ICD-9 protocols.

The training expands to 57-62 hours for all others. AHIMA indicated that most coders should receive their training three to six months prior to ICD-10 implementation so the information remains fresh in their mind.

More Codes for All

ICD-10 contains 141,000 alphanumeric codes, but all practices won't use the full complement of codes.

General physicians may use 30 more while rheumatologists and orthopedic surgeons may use up to 60 percent of the new codes. ICD-10-CM codes are used for the diagnosis and description of symptoms.

Easing the Transition

Using an EMR and computer-assisted coding will significantly reduce problems. EMRs are capable of handling all the new codes. Additionally, some systems identify potential problems and notify billers/coders before the claim leaves the office for reduced denials.

The systems still rely on human operators and will help alleviate an expected reduction in productivity the new codes will engender.

One problem that many have overlooked is a decrease in morale associated with the transition. Many coders/billers are anxious and nervous about the new coding.

Their primary concern is cash flow. The ability to maintain expected cash flow is crucial for all private practices. It's a legitimate concern and one that clinicians and billing specialists will need to work on together.

Training Opportunities

The Centers for Medicare and Medicaid Services, the World Health Organization, professional billing/coder organizations, and some insurance providers have developed training modules and tools to assist individuals in their quest for reliable training options.

Coders are the professionals that bridge the gap between clinicians and insurance companies to ensure practitioners get paid.

One of the biggest problems facing billers/coders is finding the time to learn ICD-10 coding while maintaining their typical work day with ICD-9 coding.

Online education is a convenient remedy that can be a cost effective solution for practices.

Plan for Contingencies

The best way to learn is by doing, and professional coder/biller organizations highly recommend that anyone who will be working with the new codes conduct simulations using actual claims.

The exercise provides practical experience and helps familiarize coders/billers with codes before the official rollout.

Clinicians need to establish a crisis committee to formulate a backup plan to accommodate slowdowns in reimbursements during the first few months.

The U.S. is one of the last countries to adopt the ICD-10 coding, and it's coming at a time when many practices are still involved in meeting meaningful use standards and changes associated with Obamacare.

CHAPTER 11

Minimizing Financial Havoc

The implementation of ICD-10 codes will have a financial impact on all practices. Practitioners will need to prepare for situations ranging from software errors that prevent reimbursements to the cost of staff training.

This requires a strategic plan that addresses the potential for multiple problems that will directly affect a clinic's financial security and well-being.

Maintain Cash Reserves – Plan Ahead

A practice's cash flow depends on coders/billers obtaining the best turnaround times on claims and that may not happen in the early months of ICD-10 implementation.

The reimbursement process will undoubtedly experience slow downs, and clinicians would do well to have sufficient cash reserves on hand to pay the bills and staff during the growing pains the new system is sure to suffer.

It's best to acquire a business line of credit or a business credit card with a 0% APR for six to nine months to help tide over the first few months after ICD-10 is implemented.

Training and Education Essentials – Invest in Resources

Some practice owners will be fortunate to have staff training provided by vendors. Those who aren't will be required to locate competent contractors who can provide the specialized training and education required for the implementation.

Everyone within the practice will require training. This includes the billers/coders, as well as clinicians, who will need to modify clinical documentation to justify the increased specificity with the ICD-10 coding system.

Without enough training, the bills will keep coming back to practitioners to fix, which will delay the entire payment process.

In-House or Outsourced Billing – Examine Pros and Cons

Practitioners who are considering outsourcing will want to weigh the costs of training for in-house services against hiring an outside firm to handle those duties. Coders/billers will need substantial training to minimize the disruption of reimbursements.

Experienced billers/coders are already in short supply, and it may be financially better for the practice to hire a specialist who has already undergone training.

The Impact of Security Vulnerabilities – Protect Data

Maintaining security is a very real concern, especially with the array of potential problems surrounding the transition.

Ensuring the security of patient information may include the purchase and installation of security software, while others may incur additional costs from vendors who are responsible for the system's integrity. Mistakes, oversights or compliance issues can cost a practice dearly.

Prepare for the Threat of RAC Audits – Maintain Compliant Documentation

No one wants to hear that they are the target of a Recovery Audit Contractor (RAC). ICD-10 implementation errors could appear as an attempt at fraud or abuse, causing a stain on a clinician's reputation and disruption of the practice's operation.

The best way for a clinic to prepare is for the clinician to improve their documentation standards with the increased specificity that is necessary to justify the use of the new ICD-10 codes.

An RAC intervention is a lengthy and costly process for a private practice owner. In fact, it has the potential to drive a practice out of business. The implementation of ICD-10 coding will take an economic toll on practices of all sizes. Preparing for the transition requires that clinicians use all their deductive skills to identify areas where the coding change will have an economic effect and plan for every contingency.

CHAPTER 12

Implementing EMR for ICD-10

Reality Check: Not all systems and staff are ready to transition to EMR and for the challenges your practice will face in the new age of ICD-10. The manner in which you implement is critical.

Electronic medical records will revolutionize how you run your practice and make life simpler for everyone who works in the office, from receptionists to physical therapists, as well as for your patients.

Implementing an electronic medical records system can be a little frightening. After all, you will probably be paying a fair sum of money to the vendor and you need to know that the one you have implemented is right for you.

Additionally, any transition can be difficult as everyone will need to learn new strategies and give up their old habits.

Get your team used to using hardware

Sometimes the implementation of an EMR system may fail because the team that was supposed to use the system was uncomfortable with the use of computer hardware.

If your clinic has staff members who do not know how to use a computer or aren't skilled enough to use the software they will be interacting with on a daily basis, you have some work to do. Don't assume that your staff is ready. Make sure that they are.

Analyze your workflow

There's no getting around it; an electronic medical records system is going to change how you work. You need to make sure that you – and everyone else in the office – are ready for that.

Analyze how your process currently works and talk about how it will change when you implement an EMR system. Make sure that the process makes sense. Work with the software vendor's technical staff to make sure you understand how everything is meant to work.

Input all data

EMR software is only as good as the trained users who enter the records. The objective of every single staff member of the clinic should be to become an advanced user of the EMR software.

It may take some time, but the process of including all your patient information in an EMR will mean that you move away from physical records. It is best to make sure that all information has been accounted for in order to maximise the benefit associated with EMR software.

Upgrade to the necessary hardware

This is a big one. While you can usually get away with running software on underpowered machines, it is not a good idea. You will have very little stability when using your electronic medical records software for your clinic if your computers are outdated and slow.

Assign a Project Manager or Team Leader

Usually, this position is given to the office manager or another administrative executive. No matter who does the job, it is critical that someone is responsible for pulling everything together. They will be responsible for figuring out which healthcare EMR software is best for your practice, and they will need to get buy-in from the entire staff.

They will set up a schedule for implementation and manage expectations so that nobody feels surprised or overwhelmed by the changes. They will also need to assess and do an inventory on your current resources and decide what needs to be purchased.

Include Everyone

Having a point person is crucial to implementing your EMR, and one of the most important jobs that this staff member will do is manage the expectations of the rest of the staff. One of the hardest parts of transitioning to an EMR and software is that staff members are (understandably) set in their ways and do not want to change.

Staff member buy-in should be prioritized by adding meetings or interviews to the schedule and plan. Each staff member's job should be reviewed to some degree, and the changes they will need to make should be determined and discussed in advance.

Invest in Training Programs

It is challenging and stressful for staff members to learn on the go. If your clinic is about to change the way things work, staff must be prepared.

A healthcare EMR should improve efficiency. While there will always be a bit of a lag at first, the more training given before implementation, the smoother the implementation will go.

Be Flexible

Make a schedule, ensure that the staff is ready, and transition your practice to an EMR software, but remember that there will always be challenges and the adjustment period will never be perfect. Build some flexibility into your schedule and ensure that your staff has enough time to understand ICD-10.

CHAPTER 13

EMR Implementation to Improve Workflow and Cash flow

EMR software is a significant aspect of proper preparation for ICD-10. We conclude by discussing the benefits and ways of streamlining workflow in private practice.

As healthcare continues to get competitive, the ability to cut costs and improve efficiency is essential for success. An EMR software can help your practice plan for ICD-10, in addition to several additional benefits.

<u>Some of the benefits include:</u>
- Having the ability to identify where unknown problems have crept into office procedures. Healthcare billing is quite complex. The use of electronic medical records

- Electronic medical records place a wide range of data at a clinician's fingertips to evaluate staffing needs and deploy clinicians where they are productive and efficient.

- Paperwork is destined to become obsolete with electronic medical records that store documents digitally. This will increase productivity and customer service because all medical information is easily accessible.

Electronic medical records are revolutionizing healthcare treatment by putting critical decision support systems in the hands of skilled healthcare professionals, giving them the information they need to make timely decisions.

The future of healthcare will continually keep getting better with the intelligent application of electronic medical records technology, a patient-centered focus and a dedication of trained healthcare professionals.

Easy Access to Records

With EMR software, keeping track of your patients' records is simple. Your database should be easily searchable so you can instantly pull up all the information you have on the patient, from exercise and appointment schedules to the medications they are taking.

That means no paper records to flip through, the ability to search the documents instantly for information, and no unintelligible handwritten notes. Electronic medical records are the ultimate healthcare management solution.

Compliant, Comprehensive Documentation

With electronic medical records, you can easily document everything that a patient does in real time. From the arrival to billing to the appointment itself, all information can be displayed to give you a complete record of everything about the patient.

Rapid Transmission of (and Access to) Medical Records

Sending electronic medical records using your EMR software should streamline inter-office communications. Most EMR solutions integrate seamlessly with online cloud storage, and through these cloud storage solutions you can get the records to any other healthcare provider that the patient is working with. It doesn't even matter if the other facility has integrated electronic medical records for healthcare services. You can still access the files as long as you have a computer connected to the internet.

The use of an integrated EMR software will help bring healthcare into the next century, riding practices of outdated technology and wasted energy and effort.

Streamlined, Efficient Billing

Healthcare billing can be a pain. As with all forms of accounting, keeping the information synced to the patient is difficult. Electronic medical records and healthcare documentation can make the process far more comfortable.

With a healthcare scheduling software, you can track patient visits and patient balances.

The right healthcare software makes billing patients an incredibly simple procedure and reduces the possibility of human error.

Legibility of Information

This might be the most important one. Illegible handwriting is an issue with documentation and healthcare billing.

This problem is eliminated with EMR software. All information is entered in on a computer screen, whether it is an iPad for a mobile solution or a desktop office computer. That means that all the information is well organized, printed clearly and is easy to understand. In other words, you don't have to worry about others not being able to read your handwriting.

How to Choose

For many firms, price is an important consideration, but there are times when a low price could result in fewer features and higher long-term costs. If an electronic medical record program is affordable, make sure it has everything you are looking for.

Focus on Design

Remember, you and your team are going to have to use this EMR software every day. It should be intuitive and practical. That means no excessive clicks to get through note-taking or record updates and an easy-to-understand interface.

The interface matters, because if the program isn't easy and fun to use, it will feel like more of a burden than a solution. A surprising number of electronic medical records vendors don't focus on design and usability.

Analytics is Important

You will be using your healthcare documentation software to keep track of your patients. That also means that you need to be able to use it to get information back out.

You should be able to retrieve important information about your patients – prescriptions, medical history, objective measurements, clinical assessment and patient progress.

Healthcare documentation software is only as good as its ability to quickly provide you with critical pieces of information.

Avoid Gimmicks and Sales Pitches

The goal of a salesman is to sell you a product. Although there is nothing wrong with a sales process that educates the buyer, it is important to identify the facts and ask important questions.

After all, the selection of an EMR system is one of the most important decisions you will make in your practice.

Remember to try the electronic medical records software and have as many members of your team test it out before you decide to invest.

An EMR Can Lead to Personal Freedom

Verifying Insurance Coverage

From the moment a client makes an appointment to the moment the patient encounter is completed, an EMR is on the job, increasing efficiency and boosting productivity.

An EMR has the tools to verify insurance information prior to the client's visit, providing practitioners with the information needed to formulate a treatment plan based on insurance limitations, coverage, and eligibility.

Fewer Hours and More Money

A fully integrated EMR includes a secure patient portal where individuals can complete a health history online. That information is available prior to the client's visit, allowing clinicians to familiarize themselves with the patient's problems before they arrive. The data can decrease the wait times for patients and practice owners and reduce the time spent gathering information in the exam room.

The information gathered with an EMR allows practice owners to see more patients during a typical work day and manage treatment options without the need to stay late or conduct extended hours.

24/7 Access

Patient records are updated instantly with an EMR, which can provide a single resource for all aspects of the practice's management needs. The records can be accessed from multiple locations.

If a patient requires treatment in the emergency room, the on-call clinical has all the information needed to evaluate and treat the patient without the need to contact the patient's physician.

Space and Time

Office supplies represent a significant expense for practices. An EMR saves everything digitally, eliminating the need for paper documents, files, folders and all the related products needed to manage the mountain of paperwork.

EMRs require a fraction of the space required for file cabinets to house paper records. There's no need to search and sift through dozens of documents to locate a specific paper and the technology eliminates misplaced files.

Errors and Reimbursements

With an EMR, reimbursement claims are submitted electronically in real time. The technology contains the ability to identify errors, mistakes and potential difficulties with claims before they are transmitted.

A complete record of each transaction is maintained, along with patient balances, and payments can be received in a rapid, efficient manner. EMR software helps clinicians to work smarter, not harder. The result is increased efficiency and productivity.

This helps identify documentation, billing and coding errors while reducing denials and rejections. This allows your practice to prepare for ICD-10, and setting the stage for growth at the same time.

RESOURCES

PROGRAMS FOR HEALTHCARE PROFESSIONALS

PRIVATE PRACTICE SUMMIT

PRIVATE PRACTICE SUMMIT

The world's most successful private practice owners gather for two days every year to reveal their closely guarded secrets and shortcuts rapidly to engineer a practice that thrives in the new economy.

Discover systems to get more patients, multiply revenue streams, hire staff and boost revenue with less work, frustration and stress while you regain your freedom.

To Learn More, Go To:

www.PrivatePracticeSummit.com

REFERRAL IGNITION

SCHEDULE A CALL

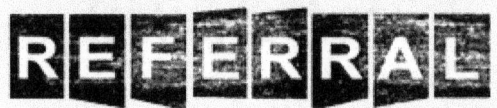

REFERRALS MADE EASY

Join the elite private practice owners who save thousands of dollars on documentation, billing, and marketing with a one-stop solution that guarantees you an endless amount of referrals for your practice.

Referral Ignition is a powerful, yet easy-to-use suite of tools that will immediately transform your practice by igniting new patient referrals, streamlining your documentation, simplifying your billing and automating follow up. It doesn't matter whether you have a website or a patient email list, are entirely new in your practice or have been in practice for 20 years with multiple clinics.

To Learn More, Go To:

www.ReferralIgnition.com

IN TOUCH BILLING SERVICE

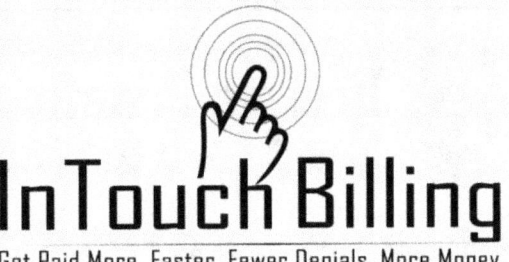

Get Paid More. Faster. Fewer Denials. More Money.

At In Touch Billing, we specialize in medical billing for all types of private practices, including rehab clinics (PT / OT / Chiropractic), speech therapy clinics and mental health clinics. We go above and beyond a 'regular billing service' because we'll give you tools to get more patients, document effectively and monitor your metrics intelligently.

We don't just bill for your practice. We help you grow your practice. With an integrated EMR and billing software, we'll save you thousands of dollars each month. In fact, a single phone call can lower your costs by as much as 20%. Call us at 800-421-8442 to learn more about the In Touch Biller Pro software and the In Touch Billing service. In most cases, we can show you how to reduce your medical billing costs.

To Learn More, Go To:
www.InTouchBilling.com

PRIVATE PRACTICE MASTERMIND

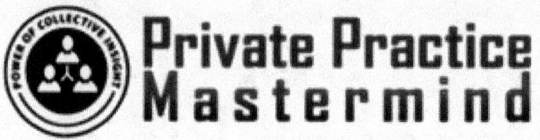

What if you could tap into the mind of the author of this book to unlock all the proven strategies that took him years to perfect? What if you could apply them within minutes to skyrocket your private practice to multiple six and even seven figure incomes for a fraction of the time, energy and cost you would typically invest... would you?

You can hire Nitin Chhoda, the "Hidden Genius" behind HUNDREDS of successful private practices, to PERSONALLY coach you to get new patients, ignite referrals from existing referral sources and reactivate former patients...

PLEASE NOTE – This exclusive coaching program is NOT for everyone. We are very selective about who we accept into the program.

To Learn More, Go To:

www.PrivatePracticeMastermind.com/

SOFTWARE FOR HEALTHCARE PROFESSIONALS
IN TOUCH EMR

Everything you need to grow your practice in on one system.

Your EMR and billing software should simplify the BEFORE, DURING and AFTER patient experience. Here's how you can streamline the 'DURING' patient experience with In Touch EMR.

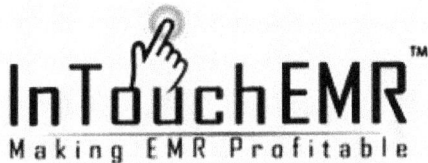

Integrated Scheduling, Documentation, Billing, and Marketing

THE DURING PATIENT EXPERIENCE
(streamlining documentation)

- Medicare compliance
- Point and click template creation
- Unlimited faxing
- Medical records upload
- Incomplete notes tracking
- Functional Limitation G codes and PQRS reporting / alerts
- Claims automatically submitted to the billing software

To Learn More, Go To:
www.InTouchEmr.com

IN TOUCH BILLER PRO

Instant transmission of claims from EMR to billing software, one click claim scrubbing, full clearing house integration, automatic posting of ERAs and seamless denial management.

Here are some of the ways in which In Touch Biller Pro boosts the efficiency of your front desk and biller:

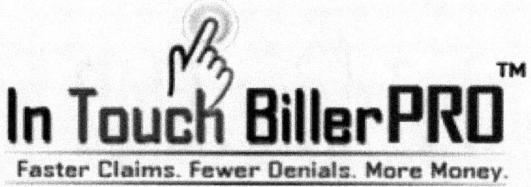

Get Paid More, Faster with Patent-Pending Billing Automation

THE BEFORE PATIENT EXPERIENCE (front desk automation)
- Online eligibility verification
- One click patient chart creation
- Automatic appointment reminders
- Automatic emailed newsletters
- Streamlined patients intake (iPad app)
- Authorization tracking and alerts
- Physician certification period tracking and alerts
- Progress note tracking and alerts

THE AFTER PATIENT EXPERIENCE (billing automation)

- Complete billing software and clearinghouse integration like you've never seen before
- Automatic claim scrubbing
- Flexibility for biller to review / edit / update claims prior to payer submission
- Auto-posting of ERAs
- Tracking patient payments (co-pays, deductibles) and patient receipt printing
- Shifting the crossover balance to secondary with one click
- Automatic batching of claims
- Streamlined denial management
- 100+ reports, completely customizable

To Learn More, Go To:

www.InTouchBillerPro.com/

THERAPY NEWSLETTER

One of the biggest challenges faced by most physical therapy private practice owners is staying in touch with patients on a regular basis. That's exactly why I created the 'Therapy Newsletter", a powerful, automated, done-for-you newsletter marketing system. Each month, we send out TWO patient newsletters to your patients and you get to choose between email, video, print and fax versions.

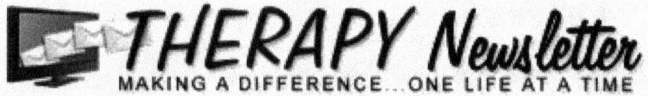

Automated Patient Newsletter (Email, Video, Print, Fax)

To Learn More, Go To:
www.TherapyNewsletter.com/

CLINICAL CONTACT

Get ready to revolutionize your patient follow-up with the power of Clinical Contact. In the new world, email and snail mail are not the only ways to reach your patients. Put the power of technology in your hands with mobile texts, voice broadcasting and email to INSTANTLY reach busy patients overwhelmed with traditional marketing messages. There's never been a faster, easier way to get more patients, engage patients and maximize retention.

Clinical Contact is the first web-based follow-up software to automate time-consuming activities for your staff. Text, voice, and email messaging with done-for-you scripts and mobile keywords open up a range of possibilities for your clinic.

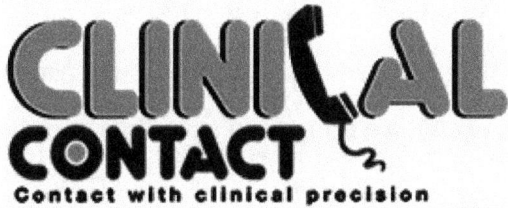

Automated Appointment Reminders with Mobile, Email, and Voice Broadcasting

To Learn More, Go To:
www.ClinicalContact.com/

SCHEDULE A CALL

I know it's challenging to work in your practice treating patients all day and marketing your clinic to increase revenue at the same time.

Are you frustrated with the painfully slow growth of referrals and high cancelation rates (despite the increasing number of evaluations)? Are you tired of declining profit margins as a direct result of hospitals and physician-owned practices?

You are probably lacking a system to ignite referrals from various sources, leaving you in the unenviable position of dependence on a handful of referral sources. Without them, your stream of incoming patients could dry up. Even after you get multiple referral sources, you need a system to motivate and train staff to "condition" patients for maximum retention and referral generation. (Just imagine if your team could transform "regular patients" into "human billboards!")

Are you just plain exhausted… from the endless hours of trying to grow your practice, spend quality time with your family and build a stable financial future all at the same time?

There is a solution.

I'd like to invite you to a strategy phone call with one of my trusted practice analysts. In this call, you will discover how to get more patients, train your staff and retain more patients... and this will not cost you a single penny.

In the live one-on-one phone call, you will learn how to:

- Get new patients
- Boost referrals from existing patients (and train your staff to do this for you)
- Gain recognition in your community

That's not all... you will also understand the different media and systems it takes to accomplish all this. At the end of this initial planning session, one of two things will happen:

1. You love the plan and decide to implement it on your own.

2. You love the plan and ask to become our client so we can personally help you execute, maximize and profit

from it. If that's the case, we'll share some information about our services.

The difference between where you are now and where you could be after scheduling this strategy call could be worth tens of thousands of dollars to your practice.

Think about it this way.

If you see 60 visits a week now and you can bump that up to 70, what would that mean? With an average reimbursement of $80 per visit, you would be looking at an additional $800 PER WEEK, which is over $40,000 a year (minimum).

What would an extra $40,000 a year (minimum) do for you?

Schedule Your Call Now:
www.StrategyCall.com

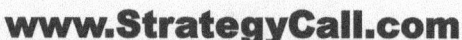

ABOUT THE AUTHOR

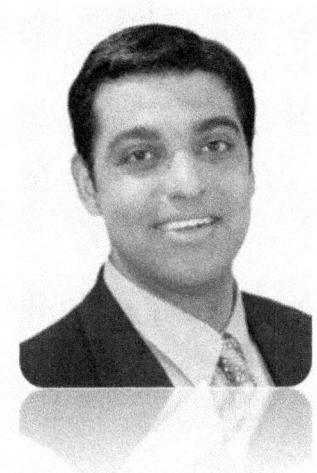

Nitin Chhoda PT, DPT, CSCS is a licensed physical therapist in NJ, NY and a published author of "Private Practice Marketing For The New Economy". He also created "Electronic Health Records and Medical Billing Software Simplified – The Before, During and After Practice Workflow".

He is also a private practice marketing consultant and just a regular guy who enjoys time with his wife (also a physical therapist) in their home in New Jersey. He enjoys techno music, watching House of Cards and Homeland. Nitin's favorite activity is writing articles, speaking at conferences and consulting with clients on the phone. He also loves to find new ways to automate marketing and referral generation using technology and, in general, juggles multiple roles as a writer, consultant, and inventor.

Nitin has written several articles on physical therapy marketing for IMPACT, ADVANCE and PT Magazine, in addition to his blog **www.nitin360.com** (a highly ranked blog on Google for physical therapy marketing). He is the founder of the **Referral Ignition training systems** and the **In Touch EMR** electronic medical records and documentation system for healthcare professionals.

He has also created the **In Touch Biller Pro** electronic billing software for healthcare professionals and the **In Touch Billing service** – affordable outsourced billing services for any healthcare practices.

He is the pioneer behind the **Private Practice Summit** in New Jersey, the **Private Practice Retreat** in Las Vegas and a mentor in the exclusive **Private Practice Mastermind** group.

He has presented on more than one occasion at the Private Practice Section Meeting of the American Physical Therapy Association. He has conducted talks at several locations in the US, Canada, and Asia.

He is also the creator of the **Therapy Newsletter** automated newsletter marketing system and **Clinical Contact**, a web-based mobile, email and voice broadcasting system. These tools help practices boost patient arrival rates and increase revenue.

Nitin is a prolific speaker and has served an adjunct faculty member on Health, Wellness and Kinesiology at Millersville University, PA. He served as a guest speaker at the annual South Asian Student's Association 2005 in Los Angeles, CA and the University of Michigan, Ann Arbor.

He was a keynote speaker at Shades of Brown, an international educational conference in Toronto, CA.

INDEX

A

AHIMA, 37

B

Billers, 25

C

claims, 2, 13, 19, 20, 21, 25, 28, 34, 39, 41, 60, 68, 69

Claims, 3, 31

clinicians, 6, 7, 12, 13, 15, 16, 17, 19, 23, 24, 25, 26, 28, 32, 33, 34, 37, 38, 39, 41, 42, 44, 52, 58, 60

Clinicians, 7, 15, 18, 21, 27, 28, 31, 40

coders, 19, 20, 25, 37, 38, 39, 41, 42, 43

Coders/billers, 42

codes, 1, 2, 3, 4, 5, 6, 7, 11, 12, 13, 15, 16, 19, 23, 25, 28, 29, 32, 33, 34, 37, 38, 39

E

Electronic Health Records and Medical Billing Software, 75

electronic medical record program, 55

electronic medical records, 46, 47, 48, 51, 52, 53, 55, 76

Electronic medical records, 46, 52, 53, 54

EMR, 2, 3, 13, 15, 16, 17, 24, 28, 38, 46, 47, 48, 49, 50, 51, 53, 54, 55, 58, 59, 60, 65, 67, 68, 76

F

fraud or abuse, 43

H

hardware, 21, 24, 27, 32, 47, 48

Health Organization and the Center for Disease Control, 4

Health, Wellness and Kinesiology, 77

healthcare, 5, 2, 3, 4, 6, 12, 17, 18, 49, 51, 52, 53, 54, 55

Healthcare, 1, 51, 54, 56

I

ICD-10, 2, 1, 2, 3, 4, 5, 6, 7, 9, 10, 11, 12, 13, 15, 16, 17, 19, 20, 21, 23, 24, 25, 26, 27, 28, 29, 31, 33, 34, 35, 37, 38, 39, 40, 41, 42, 43, 44, 46, 50, 51

ICD-10 codes, 2, 3, 4, 6, 11, 15, 16, 17, 19, 20, 21, 23, 26, 28, 29, 31, 34, 37, 41, 43

ICD-9, 1, 5, 6, 9, 10, 11, 12, 13, 15, 28, 37, 39

In Touch Biller Pro, 65, 68, 76

In Touch Billing, 65, 76

In Touch EMR, 13

insurance, 3, 6, 16, 28, 39, 58

M

medical professionals, 7

Medicare, 20, 23, 39

N

Nitin Chhoda, 3, 66, 75

O

Obamacare, 40

of ICD-9 coding, 9

outsourcing, 42

P

physical, 46, 48, 70, 75, 76

physician, 59, 72

physicians, 19, 38

practitioners, 6, 11, 12, 17, 24, 26, 31, 34, 39, 42, 58

Practitioners, 7, 15, 16, 18, 24, 27, 32, 41, 42

Private Practice, 75, 76

private practice owners, 63, 64, 70

procedure, 21, 54

R

reimbursement, 2, 3, 7, 21, 31, 34, 41, 60, 74

S

specialized, 33, 42

staff training, 3, 24, 27, 28, 32, 41, 42

staff training., 3, 24, 41

T

therapists, 3, 4, 46

training, 17, 21, 23, 25, 29, 32, 37, 39, 42, 43, 49, 76

W

World Health Organization,, 39

www.ingramcontent.com/pod-product-compliance
Lightning Source LLC
Chambersburg PA
CBHW051730170526
45167CB00002B/876